Fat Burning Foods and Recipes

Foods and Recipes That Help to Burn Fat Fast Even While You Are Resting or Sleeping

Introduction

I want to thank you and congratulate you for downloading the book, *"Fat Burning Foods and Recipes: Foods and Recipes That Help to Burn Fat Fast Even While You Are Resting or Sleeping"*.

This book contains proven steps and strategies on how to lose weight even while you are sleeping by simply eating foods that burn fat and promote overall wellness at the same time.

In this book, you will learn the reasons why you easily pack more pounds than other people, or why you are fat even when you work out and stay physically active. No two people are the same, after all, and what works for one person may not work on you. But the real highlight of this books is the foods and recipes that burn fat throughout the day and long after you sleep. By eating the foods outlined in this book and cooking the fat-burning recipes provided, you can eat without packing the pounds. Now who doesn't want that?

Thanks again for downloading this book, I hope you enjoy it!

Table of Contents

Chapter 1 – Digging Through the Fat Facts

If you bought this book, there is little doubt that you want to dig right to the good stuff. Food, after all, often plays a major role where weight loss or losing belly fat is concerned. So the idea of foods and recipes that can help you lose weight even while you're sleeping has likely caused your interest and curiosity to shoot through the roof. Imagine eating your way to a slim and slender physique, and just allowing food to do the weight lifting on your behalf.

But the truth is there are reasons that you are gaining weight, you find it more difficult to lose belly fat than any of your peers, or that you are predisposed to becoming obese. Any of these reasons could render your efforts to lose weight ineffective or a total waste of time. This is why it's very important that you understand how your body works, so you can identify which weight loss regimen will work best for you.

Fact: More than two in three adults are considered to be overweight or obese.

This data is from a 2009-2010 National Health and Nutrition Examination Survey, something that probably has changed significantly by now. Whether or not you fall in the overweight category, it is a reality that obesity is a prevailing problem in the United States and the rest of the world, and one of the most likely culprits is food, particularly the processed and fatty kind.

But what makes you fat?

While there are plenty of other factors at play, food is a major contributor to obesity. It can be caused by one of two things: either you are eating too much, or you are eating the wrong types of foods.

It is possible that vegetables rarely make it to your plate and, if it does, it is usually the starchy kind. You drink more soda than water, and you often help yourself to a second serving of everything. On top of all these, you have chronic stress and you lack sleep, resulting in you always feeling hungry and eating too much because it makes you feel better.

But why are you still fat when you've tried nearly every weight loss tips you've encountered?

It could be that the diet you are following is low fat yet highly processed. Did you consult with a dietician or nutritionist about your diet plan? If you are like most people, you probably just follow what you read.

You should also look into the possibility of hormonal imbalance, which can cause problems on your overall health and add extra pounds that you seriously don't need. Find out if you have adrenal fatigue that has a direct link to weight gain. Imbalanced hormones has a similar effect as stress and inadequate sleep.

If you're taking any medication, weight gain could be a side effect, which might explain why all your weight loss efforts are going down the drain. Speak to a health care practitioner regarding your concern. Make sure to weigh the positive and negative effects of your medication before opting to change it.

But a contradictory cause of weight gain is that you're either eating too much or eating too little. Apparently, both will lead to the same result. Eat too much and you are packing in calories. Eat too little and your body will hold on to the fat in order to survive.

Your age also has an effect on weight gain and loss. As you probably know, your metabolic rate declines as you age. Women also tend to pack in belly fat after menopause. It is a sad fact of life, but something that you can fight.

But why are you still fat when you work out?

All that exercise without any effect can be really frustrating. But it is possible that you are doing it wrong or that you choose the wrong workout. If you're trying to lose belly fat, for example, running on a treadmill for hours would not be enough to trim your waist. You should to a combination of training, such as weights and cardio workouts.

Well, no one will blame you if you want to reach for that double cheeseburger after reading this, but you should seriously reconsider. There is no need to starve yourself, but you should choose to eat healthy and slim.

Chapter 2 – Eating Your Way to a Slim and Healthy Body

There is something about processed and fatty foods that make them irresistible and, in some cases, make you quite happy and satisfied. If not for the fatty repercussions, it would be very nice to pack your fridge with them. Since this is not the case, it is best to start changing your diet into something that promotes overall wellness, a longer life, and a fit body.

Fat-Burning Food That Does Wonders Even While You Sleep

Late-night snackers rejoice! There are now food and recipes that burn fat even when you are sound asleep and snoring with gusto. For a lot of people, this is like a dream come true. After all, the usual advice is to eat early and avoid midnight snacks, something you can't help to disobey if you are working late. It is often a case of what the stomach wants the stomach should get.

Well, no more depriving yourself of what will make you happy and your tummy satisfied. To keep the weight off, however, you need to choose your foods wisely. What is great about most fat-burning foods is that they burn more calories than what they contain. So if you eat them all throughout the day, not just during dinner or before you go to sleep, your body will continue to burn calories for 24 hours.

Are you ready to start eating?

Whole Grains

Barley, quinoa, spelt, wheat bran, kamut, wheat germ, brown rice and whole wheat contain nutrients that help keep your insulin levels low, burning fat in the process. These are also a rich source of fiber and complex carbohydrates that are essential in stimulating your metabolism, resulting in more calories and fat burned. Think it's too late night to raid the fridge and whip up something? Eating a whole grain fruit-filled bar before bed will give your body the boost to burn calories while you snooze.

Fish

Fish contains Omega 3 that not only keeps your heart healthy, but also helps in weight loss. As it happens, deficiency in Omega 3 results in insufficient sleep that can lead to unhealthy late-night eating. This has something to do with the pineal gland in your brain that is responsible for regulating your nervous system. It needs Omega 3 to function properly and the deficiency of it results in changes in the production of the sleep hormone melatonin, which leads to restless rather than restful nights.

In addition, fish is rich in protein, which burns more calories when digested compared to digesting fats or carbs. It will also keep you feeling full for a longer period, effectively curbing the hunger pangs. It is also low in fat and calories. So even if you're not a big fan, you might want to start liking it for the sake of a fit and healthy body.

To get the most out of fish, it is best to grill, bake or broil it, instead of frying it. Salmon and tuna are quite fatty for fish standards, but they are just as nutritious and beneficial, just make sure you stick to 3 ounces of serving in every meal. Other highly recommended types are halibut, wild salmon and Pacific cod. For variety, you can substitute fish with oysters or scallops.

Legumes

Legumes, such as lentils, split peas and other bean varieties, is generally healthy but they also have downsides, which is why they have become quite controversial. Legumes is your source of plant-based dietary protein and fiber — highly nutritious and very affordable. Unfortunately, raw legumes contain anti-nutrients, substances that interfere with absorption of other nutrients and digestion. But you can take them out of the equation by following the proper methods of preparing legumes, such as soaking, sprouting and boiling them.

Milk

There may be a lot of contradictions when it comes to dairy foods, but milk has been proven to boost weight loss. As a rich source of mineral calcium, it can break down fat cells that are responsible for your added weight, but you need to consume anywhere between 1200 and 1300 mg daily. Milk also contains complex carbohydrate that keep insulin levels low. This helps boost metabolism and burns calories. Drink skim milk to get maximum benefits without the added calories.

Are you lactose-intolerant by any chance or have allergies with anything dairy related? You can still get calcium from other sources, such as broccoli, bok choy, collard greens, canned salmon, edamame, figs and sardines.

Citrus fruits

The best citrus fruits to consume to help you lose weight while sleeping should not only contain vitamin C, but also fiber. Both essential elements can be found in grapefruit, oranges, papaya, tomatoes, limes, lemons and tangerines. Whether you eat them or drink their juice, you will surely see a change on the weighing scale, because of the carnitine amino acid in vitamin C that will stimulate the fat-burning capability of your body. It dilutes fat and then eliminates it from your body. Fiber, on the other hand, will increase metabolism and burn fat.

Cherries

Who doesn't love cherries, especially when topped on your favorite cocktail or dessert? If you take out the fattening elements and simply munch on plenty of cherries, you can enjoy a delicious way to burn belly fat. Cherries can raise the melatonin levels in your body, which is responsible for promoting a good night's sleep. And you know what they say about a restful night — no hunger pangs throughout the day. It is also a powerful antioxidant that leaves little doubt of its ability to promote weight loss.

Nuts

Nuts may belong to the legumes family, but it deserves a spot of its own what with its many benefits that includes burning fat. One of its positive effects have a direct connection with a peaceful and good night's sleep brought on by the magnesium that is present in nuts. When you're sleeping better, you do not overeat and gain weight. Women who eat nuts are also at a lower risk of dangerous inflammation, a reaction of the immune system that could lead to heart disease diabetes, Alzheimer's disease or cancer.

Some of the best nuts for your diet include almonds, pistachios and cashews, while the best nuts for your heart and brain are walnuts and peanuts, respectively. When buying pre-packaged nuts, make sure it only contains 100 to 200 calories per pack.

There are plenty of other fat-burning foods out there, but these are the easiest to find and ones that you would normally stock up in your home. So why not whip up a mix of cherries and nuts before you go to bed? Or, you can take note of different recipes that will help burn fat while you sleep.

Chapter 3 – Fat-Burning Recipes

When it comes to fat burning food, the rule of thumb is to eat the whole natural kinds that are high in vitamins and minerals but low in artificial sugar, cholesterol, saturated fat, sodium and trans fat. Guided by the list of fat-burning foods from the previous chapter and the recipes below, you can eat and sleep your way to a healthy and fit you.

Grilled Chicken Cutlets with Summer Succotash

Ingredients

1 pound of boneless chicken cutlets

1/4 tsp of salt and pepper for seasoning

1 cup of thawed lima beans

1/2 cup of corn

1/2 pint of red tomatoes

1/2 cup fresh basil leaves

1 tbsp of grated parmesan

1 tbsp olive oil

Cooking Directions

1. Slice chicken cutlets into 4 thin strips and season with salt and pepper.

2. Put grilling pan over high heat and grill chicken until it is cooked through, turning one side after 3 to 4 minutes.

3. Put a skillet on high heat and add 1 tablespoon of olive oil.

4. Add the lima beans, corn and red tomatoes.

5. Stir all the ingredients for 3 to 4 minutes or until the tomatoes burst.

6. Stir in grated parmesan and add fresh basil leaves. Tear leaves into small pieces if they are large.

7. Serve the grilled chicken with the lima beans mixture. Pair it with lemon wedges and a small whole wheat roll.

Fresh Burrito Bowl

Ingredients

3 ounces precooked grilled chicken breast thinly sliced

1/4 cup black beans

1/2 cup red cabbage thinly sliced

1 tsp chicken broth

2 tbsp nonfat Greek yogurt

2 tbsp fresh salsa

Pinch of cumin

Pinch of cayenne

Pinch of garlic powder

Fresh cilantro

Sliced green onions

Cooking Directions

1. Heat black beans with chicken broth, and then add oregano, cayenne, cumin, and garlic powder. You can also microwave the mixture on high for 30 to 45 seconds or until it is heated. Set aside.

2. In a bowl, add red cabbage into the heated mixture, and spoon the back beans on top.

3. Layer the sliced chicken, add Greek yogurt and salsa, and garnish with cilantro and green onions.

4. Serve and enjoy immediately.

BBQ Turkey Burgers

<u>Ingredients</u>

1 pound dark-meat turkey, grounded

1 clove of garlic, minced

4 slices sweet onion, grilled

1/2 tsp paprika

1/4 tsp ground cumin

1/4 tsp freshly ground black pepper

1/4 cup barbecue sauce

Pinch of kosher salt

4 (1.6 oz) sesame seed buns, toasted

<u>Cooking Directions</u>

1. Mix together turkey cumin, garlic and paprika in a bowl.

2. Form 4-inch turkey patties and season with salt and pepper.

3. Cook patties over grill heated to medium high until they are cooked through or about 7 minutes. Turn once and cook for another 7 minutes.

4. Assemble your burger with toasted sesame buns, then serve with desired toppings.

Healthy and Spicy Cauliflower Lasagna

<u>Ingredients</u>

1 1/2 pounds of 3/4 of a medium head cauliflower

7 to 8 ounces no-boil lasagna

2 tbsps extra-virgin olive oil

2 tsp red pepper flakes

2 tbsps vegetable or chicken stock

8 ounces ricotta cheese

3 cups marinara sauce

1 cup freshly grated Parmesan

Salt and freshly ground pepper

Pinch of cinnamon

<u>Cooking Directions</u>

1. Preheat the oven to 450° F

2. Clean and prepare the cauliflower, then cut each into 1/3-inch thick slices. Let the florets on the edges fall off.

3. Toss all of the cauliflower with olive oil salt and pepper

4. Line a baking sheet with parchment paper, and then place the cauliflower mixture in an even layer.

5. Roast for about 15 minutes, but when the timer hits 8 minutes, stir and flip over the big slices until they are tender. The florets should be nicely browned as well.

6. Remove cauliflowers from the oven and toss in the red pepper flakes. Set aside.

7. Turn the oven down to 350° F

8. In a bowl, mix the ricotta cheese, vegetable or chicken stock, cinnamon, and then add salt and pepper to taste. Set aside.

9. Oil a baking dish and spread a spoonful of tomato sauce. Add a layer of lasagna noodles on top. Add a layer of the ricotta cheese mixture. Top it with a layer of cauliflower, layer of tomato sauce on top, and add a layer of parmesan.

10. Repeat the layers, but end with a layer of lasagna noodles topped with tomato sauce and Parmesan.

11. With a foil, cover the baking dish tightly and then place it in the oven. Bake for 40 minutes or until the noodles are tender and the mixture bubbles.

12. Bake for another 10 minutes or until the top starts to brown, if you so desire.

13. Remove from the heat and let it sit for 5 minutes.

14. Serve with freshly cut parsley on top.

Middle Eastern Rice Salad

Ingredients

3 cups cooked brown rice

1 can (16 oz)/chickpeas, rinsed and drained

About 3/4 cup sweet onion or Vidalia, thinly sliced

2 tbsp olive oil

1/2 tsp ground cumin

1/2 cup chopped pitted dates

1/4 tsp salt

1/4 cup chopped fresh mint

1/4 cup chopped fresh parsley

Freshly ground black pepper

Cooking Directions

1. In a large skillet, heat oil over medium high heat. Add and cook onions for about 5 minutes or until it begins to brown. Remember to stir often.

2. Remove from heat and then stir in chickpeas, salt and cumin. Season with freshly ground black pepper.

3. In a large bowl, add in brown rice, onion and chickpeas mixture, mint, dates and parsley. Toss, until everything is well-combined and then serve.

Brown Rice Sushi Bowl

<u>Ingredients</u>

For Sushi Bowl:

4 cups cooked brown rice, preferably short green

2 cups mixed salad greens

6 oz sushi-grade albacore tuna dice

10 grape tomatoes, cut in half

1/3 English cucumber, diced

1/2 cup shelled edamame

1/4 cup prepared sushi vinegar or rice wine vinegar

1 small navel orange

Sesame seeds for garnish (optional)

For Dressing:

1/4 cup fresh orange juice

3 tbsps light-colored (usukushi) soy sauce

1 1/2 tsp extra virgin olive oil

1 tsp freshly grated ginger

1 tsp honey

<u>Cooking Directions</u>

1. Mix the sushi vinegar and the brown rice using a cutting motion with a flat wooden panel or a spatula. Do not stir so the rice grains won't be mashed. Cover and set aside.

2. Peel and pith off the orange, cut crosswise in slices, and then cut the slices into cubes.

3. Prepare the dressing by whisking all the ingredients in a bowl until the honey is dissolved.

4. In a large bowl, combine oranges, grape tomatoes, diced cucumber, shelled edamame and the Albacore tuna. Add the dressing and toss until well combined.

5. Place equal measures of the brown sushi rice in four bowls. In each bowl, place one quarter of the salad greens on top of the rice, and one quarter of the Albacore mixture on the other side. Serve and garnish with sesame seeds, if you so desire.

Chicken Cacciatore

Ingredients

2 8-ounce chicken breast, boneless and skinless

8 ounces mushrooms, quartered

1 14-ounce can no-salt-added diced tomatoes, drained

1 small onion, sliced

1 cup reduced-sodium chicken broth

3/4 cup sliced jarred roasted red peppers, rinsed

1/2 cup dry white wine

1/4 cup all-purpose flour

2 tablespoons extra-virgin olive oil, divided

2 teaspoons chopped fresh rosemary or 3/4 teaspoon dried

1/4 teaspoon salt, divided

1/4 teaspoon freshly ground pepper

1/4 cup quartered Kalamata olives

Cooking Directions

1. Cut each chicken breast to make 4 roughly equal portions. Season with salt and pepper and then dredge in the flour.

2. In a large skillet, heat 1 tablespoon of oil over medium heat. Cook the chicken until brown or about 2 minutes per side. Transfer to a plate and set aside.

3. In the same skillet, add remaining 1 tablespoon of oil and then throw in the mushrooms, rosemary, onion and salt. Stir frequently until the onion has softened or become

golden brown. Add in the vegetables and the rest of the flour, cook and stir until everything is coated.

4. Add wine and cook for 1 minute, while stirring all throughout. Toss in drained tomatoes, roasted red peppers, olives and broth. Let it simmer over medium-low heat.

5. Add the chicken into the pan and continue cooking for 10 minutes more or until the broth has slightly thickened and the chicken is cooked through. Serve and garnish with rosemary, if desired.

Greek Quinoa and Avocados

<u>Ingredients</u>

1/2 cup uncooked quinoa

2 avocados, pitted, peeled, and sliced

1 cup water

2 Roma (plum) tomatoes, seeded and finely chopped

1/3 cup finely chopped red onion

1/3 cup crumbled feta cheese

1/2 cup shredded fresh spinach

2 tbsps lemon juice

2 tbsps olive oil

1/2 tsp salt

Spinach leaves

<u>Cooking Directions</u>

1. In a small saucepan, add quinoa and water, and bring to a boil. Lower heat, cover and let it simmer for 15 minutes or until liquid is absorbed.

2. Transfer the mixture in a medium bowl and stir in onions, tomatoes and spinach. Set aside.

3. Whisk together oil salt and lemon juice in a small bowl. Add to the quinoa mixture.

4. On a plate, place spinach, avocado slices and the quinoa mixture. Serve with a sprinkle of grated feta cheese.

Maple Salmon with Greens, Edamame and Walnuts

<u>Ingredients</u>

4 5-ounce fresh or frozen skinless salmon fillets, about 1 inch thick

1 6-ounce package fresh baby spinach

1/2 cup cooked shelled edamame

1/2 cup red bell pepper strips

1/4 cup chopped walnuts, toasted

3 tbsps pure maple syrup

2 tbsps balsamic vinegar

2 tbsps olive oil

1 tbsps Dijon mustard

1 tbsps finely chopped shallot

2 tsps snipped fresh rosemary

1 tsp lemon juice

1/4 tsp salt

1/4 tsp freshly ground black pepper

<u>Cooking Directions</u>

1. Preheat boiler, but remove rack.

2. In a small saucepan, mix together vinegar, maple syrup, mustard, lemon juice, shallot, salt and pepper.

3. Prepare the dressing by mixing together olive oil and 2 tablespoons of the maple syrup mixture in a small bowl. Set aside.

4. Prepare the glaze by heating the remaining maple syrup mixture to a boil. Reduce heat, uncover and let it simmer until syrupy or about 5 minutes. Remove from heat and add in rosemary.

5. In a large bowl, combine edamame, spinach, nuts and pepper strips. Drizzle over the dressing and toss to coat all ingredients.

6. Place salmon on the greased, unheated rack, brush with half the glaze, and place 6 to 7 inches from heat in a preheated boiler. Broil for 5 minutes, turn over and brush with the remaining glaze. Broil some more for 3 to 5 minutes, or until fish begins to flake when tested with a fork.

7. Spoon the salad on a plate and then topped with the broiled salmon.

Tuscan Spinach, Bean & Sausage Soup

Ingredients

1 link hot Italian-style turkey sausage

1 19-ounce can cannellini beans, rinsed

1 14-ounce can reduced-sodium chicken broth

8 ounces frozen cut-leaf spinach

1 clove garlic, minced

2 tablespoons freshly grated Parmesan cheese

1/4 teaspoon dried marjoram

Salt & freshly ground pepper, to taste

Cooking Directions

1. In a small skillet, bring to a simmer over medium heat ¼-inch of water and sausage. Cook uncovered for 5 to 10 minutes or until water evaporates. Continue cooking until sausage is brown on all sides. When cool enough to handle, cut into pieces of ½-inch thick.

2. In a medium saucepan, combine broth, sliced sausages, beans, spinach, marjoram and garlic. Cover and cook for 10 minutes over medium heat. Add salt and pepper to taste. Stir in cheese right before serving.

Chapter 4 – Boost Your Metabolism

Even when you're eating fat-burning food, it pays to boost your metabolism. The combination will put your weight loss at a high speed. How do you achieve this through the way you eat?

Make sure to eat breakfast

Breakfast is not called the most important meal of the day for nothing. Your metabolism becomes idle at night and will only be switched at high speed when you enjoy your morning meal. This is because your level of cortisol is highest just before you get up in the morning, and when you eat breakfast, your body will be more than ready to turn those calories into muscles fast. As this is the only time of the day that such a phenomenon happens, you should take advantage of it by eating a morning meal.

Don't skip any meals

Some fad or crash diets may recommend that you skip breakfast or dinner, and then eat a lot at one particular meal. Doing so can throw your metabolism off balance, causing it to rev up at one point and then slow to a crawl at another. The only way to keep your engine and energy running is to eat 3 times a day with healthy meals that only have 300 to 400 calories. Experts also suggest that you snack twice a day with foods that have 200 to 300 calories.

Have your fill of smart foods

Protein takes more calories to digest, making it one of the best weight loss foods. But because you need other items that are nutritious and packed with vitamins and minerals, you must have a smart menu throughout the day. Start with a low fat turkey bacon and a piece of whole grain toast for breakfast, chicken and salad for lunch, and salmon for dinner. Eat walnuts for your snacks. You should also enjoy a dose of caffeine twice a day to accelerate the fat-burning process.

Avoid partying too hard

Study shows that bouts of heavy drinking have a direct link to excessive abdominal fat. According to the medical director of Cederquist Comprehensive Medical Weight Control in Naples, Florida, Caroline Cederquist, "With heavy alcohol intake, your body prioritizes the detoxification of the alcohol over the metabolism of fat", which means your body will hold on to the fat in exchange for detoxification.

On top of these, you should stay physically active, cut back on sugar, manage stress and go to bed early.

Conclusion

Thank you again for downloading this book!

I hope this book was able to help you to get started on your weight loss efforts, inspiring you to eat right and healthy.

The next step is to follow all the tips provided, especially the recipes so you can get rid of those excess fats and enjoy a longer and healthier existence, while you eat.

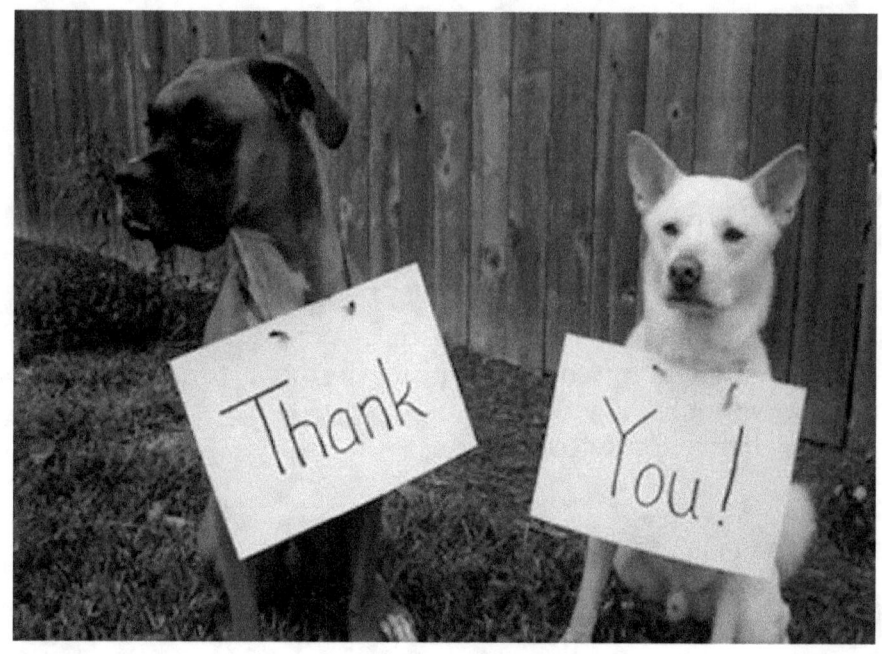

Finally, if you enjoyed this book, then I'd like to ask you for a favor, would you be kind enough to leave a review for this book on Amazon? It'd be greatly appreciated!

Click here to leave a review for this book on Amazon!

http://www.amazon.com/gp/product/B0116DMBFG

Thank you and good luck!